The Clean Eating Gout Diet & Cookbook

Improve your Gout One Meal at a Time with Low-Purine Meals

Genevieve Marchand

The Clean Eating Gout Diet & Cookbook

Copyright © 2016 by Genevieve Marchand

All rights reserved.

No part of this publication may be reproduced, distributed, or transmitted in any form or by any means, including photocopying, recording, or other electronic or mechanical methods, without the prior written permission of the publisher, except in the case of brief quotations embodied in critical reviews.

While the publisher and author have used their best efforts in preparing this book, they make no representations or warranties with respect to the accuracy or completeness of the content of this book. The material in this book is for informational purposes only. Since each individual situation is unique, you should use proper discretion, in consultation with a health-care practitioner, before undertaking the diet and strategies described in this book.

No warranty may be created or extended by the contributors/ authors, either implicitly or explicitly. The author and publisher expressly disclaim responsibility for any adverse effects that may result from the use or application of the information contained in this book.

Neither the publisher, nor contributors / authors shall be liable for any damages, including but not limited to special, incidental, consequential, or other damages.

The Clean Eating Gout Diet & Cookbook

Table of Contents

Introduction	iv
Chapter 1: Gout Explained	1
Chapter 2: What to Avoid	5
Chapter 3: Clean Eating Rules of the Road	7
Chapter 4: Breakfast	9
Chapter 5: Salads	17
Chapter 6: Soups & Appetizers	25
Chapter 7: Chicken	36
Chapter 8: Turkey	44
Chapter 9: Fish	51
Chapter 10: Meatless	58
Chapter 11: Desserts	66
Conclusion	75

Introduction

We are what we eat.

This book is about the intersection of gout and diet. More specifically, it is about incorporating clean eating habits to ward off gout.

Choosing to eat clean means filling your plate with natural, wholesome foods and excluding anything processed or refined. The idea is not deprivation, but rather rediscovering and embracing fresh, unaltered food that nourishes your body.

Utilizing a clean eating approach that eliminates processed foods and additives from your diet, we have compiled a vast array of low purine, gout friendly food and meal options that cover everything from Breakfast to Dessert that have proven to be beneficial in maintaining a healthy gout free lifestyle.

In recent years, there's been an explosion of gout. Simply put, the more obese we become as a nation, the more instances of gout and it crippling effects. Arguably, this rise is being driven by our increasing sedentary lifestyles coupled with our intake of processed food. In the last half century alone, the condition has more than doubled. Along with obesity and hypertension, rates have steadily climbed. It now affects more than 8 million American adults and the numbers keep climbing.

What do we do about it? The short answer is that we have to eat better.

The Clean Eating Gout Diet & Cookbook

As a nutritionist charged with the care of my husband who has Gout, I can safely say that it is no laughing matter. In fact, doctors say that next to childbirth and kidney stones, a gout attack is one of the most painful things a person can experience.

Gout is a form of arthritis caused by high concentration of uric acid in the blood. This leads to the formation of tiny needle like crystals in the joints and kidneys (where they form kidney stones) and less commonly in other parts of the body including the spinal cord and the vocal chords. Gout is as painful as rheumatoid arthritis.

Left untreated or uncontrolled, gout can form chalky lumps called tophi, which can severely damage joints, making walking and using the hands extremely painful. In extreme cases, joint replacements and even amputation can be necessary.

With this as our starting point, embracing a 'clean eating' diet to help prevent gout doesn't mean that you have to have a very restrictive diet, but rather embrace a 'clean eating' lifestyle that will have enumerable health benefits such as gout minimization, prevention and control.

Chapter 1: Gout Explained

Gout is a rheumatic condition that manifests itself through recurrent attacks of acute inflammatory arthritis—a red, tender, hot, swollen joint. Although gout can occur in any joint of your body and in multiple joints simultaneously, the joint at the base of the big toe, the metatarsal-phalangeal joint, is where it typically strikes.

Gout occurs when too much of a substance called uric acid builds up in the blood; this condition is also called hyperuricemia- elevated levels of uric acid in the blood. Uric acid can come from the breakdown of old cells and from certain foods and drinks. If too much uric acid is produced, or if it isn't properly excreted, it can form tiny crystals that are deposited in joints, tendons, and surrounding tissues. For this reason, gout is called a "crystal deposit disease." It may also present as tophi, kidney stones, or urate nephropathy – a kidney disease.

Essentially it is a breakdown of the metabolic process that controls the amount of uric acid in your blood. The stiffness and swelling are a result of excess uric acid forming crystals in your joints, and the pain associated with this disease is caused by your body's inflammatory response to the crystals.

What Are the Symptoms of Gout?

A gout attack, or "flare", usually strikes suddenly, and generally at night. Mysteriously, it often targets the large joint of your big toe. Your skin becomes red, inflamed, and overly sensitive. Even the light pressure of a bed sheet can become unbearable. A fever may also be present.

The pain associated with gout is often sudden and intense. Joints tend to swell, and can be warm to the touch. The skin around the joint may also take on a deep red or purple hue.

People who have had gout for extended periods of time may develop nodules beneath the skin near joints; these are accumulations of uric acid crystals. Attacks can recur in the same joint over weeks, months or years, and repeated bouts of gout can damage the joint. Kidney damage can also occur.

Gout Diagnosis

The true determinant of gout comes with a test to look for the hallmark sign of gout: uric acid crystals.

Visiting your doctor during an attack can ensure an accurate diagnosis. By drawing joint fluid during an acute attack the doctor can identify the uric acid crystals. The fluid is examined under a microscope with special filters so the crystals, if there are any, show up.

Other tests that can be used are blood tests to determine your respective uric acid level, x-rays to rule out other perceived causes of the inflammation, ultrasound to detect urate crystals in the joint or tophus and a CT scan be used to detect urate crystals in a joint. This last method is seldom used, however, due to cost.

Treatment of Gout?

There is no known cure for gout, but it can be alleviated through a variety of conventional therapies and gout treatments. During attacks, along with ice packs, physicians often prescribe non-steroidal anti-inflammatory drugs **(NSAIDs)** such as ibuprofen to keep inflammation and pain under control. **Corticosteriods** can have a similar affect; these are administered via pills or injections. Lastly, Your doctor may recommend **colchicine**(Colcrys, Mitigare), a type of pain reliever that effectively reduces gout pain and inflammation.

After an acute gout attack resolves, your doctor may prescribe a low daily dose of colchicine to prevent future attacks. There are also medicines that can lower levels of uric acid by blocking its production, the best known is probably **allopurinol** (Aloprim, Lopurin, Zyloprim) or the newer **febuxostat** (Uloric). Lastly, **Probenecid** (Probalan) improves your kidneys' ability to remove uric acid from your body. This may lower your uric acid levels and reduce your risk of gout, but the level of uric acid in your urine is increased.

Diet and Lifestyle Changes

Medications are the most proven, effective way to treat gout symptoms. However, making certain diet and lifestyle changes also may help, such as:

- Limiting alcoholic beverages and drinks sweetened with fruit sugar (fructose).
- Limit intake of foods high in purines, such as red meat, organ meats and seafood.
- Exercising regularly and losing weight. Keeping your body at a healthy weight reduces your risk of gout. Exercise increases circulation and normalizes your uric acid levels by way of mormalizing your insulin levels.
- Drink plenty of water.

Other Recommendations

If you want to investigate some alternative routes to gout prevention certain foods, vitamins and spices have been shown to minimize gout. Some such as **coffee, vitamin c, cherries** have been shown to lower uric acid levels. Others such as **apple cider vinegar** and **baking soda** have proven themselves out by making the body more on more alkaline.

Pineapples (Bromelain), beet juice and **turmeric** have also seen much favor. Pineapples contain powerful enzymes that are frequently recommended for gout. Beet juice helps prevent acidosis by stimulating the liver to cleanse the bile ducts. Lastly, turmeric has been gaining popularity in the last couple of years as a remedy for gout. It is used to reduce inflammation and oxidative stress.

Chapter 2: What to Avoid

A gout friendly approach should fundamentally start with:

- Limiting/ avoiding alcoholic beverages and drinks sweetened with fruit sugar (fructose).
- Limiting/ avoiding intake of foods high in purines, such as red meat, organ meats and seafood.

Alcohol disrupts the removal of uric acid from the body. It's thought that high levels of purine in alcoholic beverages leads to this disruption. While the breakdown of purines into uric acid would normally be flushed out of the body through the urine, this process is interrupted when uric acid levels get too high.

Fructose-rich beverages, like soft drinks, have been shown to increase the risk of developing gout. While these types of drinks don't have high amounts of purines, they do contain significant amounts of fructose — which increases uric acid levels.

Foods that are high in purines should entirely be eliminated. People with gout don't process purines well. Complications occur when the kidneys don't get rid of uric acid fast enough, or if there is an increased amount of uric acid production. These high levels build up in the blood, leading to what is known as hyperuricemia.

High Purines

All of these foods have a high purine content. With that in mind, a gout diet should avoid or limit these foods: **organ meats, brain, sweetbreads, heart, kidney, liver, beef, pork, lamb, herring, anchovies, mackerel, mussels, smelt, sardines, scallops, lobster and yeast & beer.**

Moderate Purines

Now, we move in to an area that I refer to as 'Sometime Foods' which are moderately high in purines. These foods that are somewhat high should be eaten in moderation: **grouse, mutton, bacon, salmon, turkey, partridge, trout, goose, haddock and pheasant.**

Refined Carbs

You should seek to avoid and limit refined carbs. Refined carbohydrates include: **white bread, cakes, candy, pasta (except for whole grain).**

Foods to Include Daily

You are allowed to eat the following on a daily basis: **beans and lentils, legumes, fluids, especially water, low-fat or fat-free dairy (16-24 oz daily, max), whole grains (like oats, brown rice, and barley), quinoa, sweet potatoes and fruits and vegetables.**

Chapter 3: Clean Eating Rules of the Road

Clean eating is about limiting processed and refined foods from your diet and substituting with wholefoods instead.

Incorporating a gout friendly diet with the clean eating lifestyle couldn't be easier. You just have to follow the guidelines set out below. Are they stuck in cement? No. You can have cheat days. You can set up once a week for your cheat day. I always use Fridays myself. I love pizza.

That being said, here are some of the general tenets for clean eating:

Avoid processed foods – these types of foods are usually high in additives and chemicals, salt and refined sugar and that's not something you want in your system so avoiding these foods is the best thing to do.

Avoid refined foods – this includes refined flour, sugars and fats. Cutting these down from your diet will produce weight loss and correct the insulin levels and consequently uric acid levels at the same time.

Avoid alcohol – alcohol goes into the blood which then goes into your system, disturbing the way your liver, heart or kidneys work so alcohol. Alcohol impedes the body's ability to remove uric acid.

Avoid preservatives – read the labels of each food you buy and if there's ingredients that you can barely pronounce, don't buy it! As simple as that!

Avoid artificial sweeteners – refined sugar is a no-no, but so are artificial sweeteners so don't fool yourself that you get away with it. As their name states, they are artificial, made by humans in a lab, there's nothing natural or healthy about them.

You and your food needs are important – choose your foods wisely and tailor your eating habits to suit your needs, according to your health, your daily tasks or cravings. Clean eating is a highly customizable lifestyle, keep that in mind all the time!

Establish goals and eat accordingly – losing weight or maintaining a healthy weight, fix a health problem or prevent one, clean eating can make it

Chapter 4: Breakfast

Old Fashioned Scrambled Eggs

Ingredients

- 8 eggs
- 1(5 ounce) can evaporated milk
- 2 tablespoons butter
- salt and pepper for taste

Directions

1. In a bowl, whisk the eggs and milk until combined.
2. In a skillet, heat butter until hot.
3. Add egg mixture; cook and stir over medium-low heat until eggs are completely set.
4. Season with salt and pepper.

Baked Apple Oatmeal

Ingredients

- 2 2/3 cups old-fashioned oats
- ½ cup raisins
- 4 cups milk
- 1/3 cup packed brown sugar
- 2 tablespoons butter or margarine, melted
- 1 teaspoon ground cinnamon
- ¼ teaspoon salt
- 2 medium apples, chopped (2 cups)

Directions

1. 1 Heat oven to 350°F. In 2-quart casserole, mix oats, raisins, 4 cups milk, the brown sugar, butter, cinnamon, salt and apples.
2. 2 Bake uncovered 40 to 45 minutes or until most liquid is absorbed. Top with walnuts. Serve with additional milk.

Zucchini & Eggs

Ingredients

- 4 eggs, lightly beaten
- 2 tablespoons grated Parmesan cheese
- 2 tablespoons olive oil
- 1 zucchini, sliced 1/8- to 1/4-inch thick
- garlic powder or salt
- ground black pepper to taste

Directions

1. Stir the eggs and Parmesan cheese together in a bowl; set aside.
2. Heat the olive oil in a large skillet over medium-high heat; cook the zucchini in the hot oil until softened and lightly browned, about 7 minutes. Season the zucchini with garlic powder, salt, and pepper. Reduce heat to medium; pour the egg mixture into the skillet. Cook, stirring gently, for about 3 minutes.
3. Remove the skillet from the heat and cover. Keep covered off the heat until the eggs set, about 2 minutes more and serve.

Morning Green Smoothie

Ingredients

- 1 cucumber, sliced
- 2 kiwi fruits, peeled and sliced
- 1 cup baby spinach
- 1 cup coconut milk
- 2 tablespoons raw honey
- 1 pinch ground ginger

Directions

1. Combine all the ingredients in a blender and pulse until smooth and creamy.
2. Pour the mixture into glasses and serve right away.

Cinnamon Carrot Baked Oatmeal

Ingredients

- 2 cups rolled oats
- ¼ teaspoon cinnamon powder
- ¼ teaspoon ground ginger
- ½ cup walnuts, chopped
- 2 carrots, grated
- ¼ cup maple syrup
- ¼ cup dates, pitted and chopped
- 2 cups coconut milk
- 2 tablespoons raw honey

Directions

1. Combine all the ingredients in a deep dish baking pan.
2. Cook in the preheated oven at 350F for 10-15 minutes until softened.

3. Serve the oatmeal warm.

Mom's Eggs Benedict

Ingredients

- 4 slices Canadian bacon
- 1 teaspoon white vinegar
- 4 eggs
- 1 cup butter
- 3 egg yolks
- 1 tablespoon heavy cream
- 1 dash ground cayenne pepper
- ½ teaspoon salt
- 1 tablespoon lemon juice
- 4 whole wheat English muffins, split and toasted

Directions

1. In a skillet over medium-high heat, fry the Canadian bacon on each side until evenly browned.
2. Fill a large saucepan with about 3 inches water, and bring to a simmer. Pour in the vinegar. Carefully break the 4 eggs into the water, and cook 2 to 3 minutes, until whites are set but yolks are still soft. Remove eggs with a slotted spoon.
3. Meanwhile, melt the butter until bubbly in a small pan or in the microwave. Remove from heat before butter browns.
4. In a blender or large food processor, blend the egg yolks, heavy cream, cayenne pepper, and salt until smooth. Add half of the hot butter in a thin steady stream, slow enough so that it blends in at least as fast as you are pouring it in. Blend in the lemon juice using the same method, then the remaining butter.

5. Place open English muffins onto serving plates. Top with 1 slice Canadian bacon and 1 poached egg. Drizzle with the cream sauce, and serve at once.

Pumpkin Pancakes

Ingredients

- 1 ¼ cups all-purpose flour
- 2 tablespoons sugar
- 2 teaspoons baking powder
- ½ teaspoon cinnamon
- ½ teaspoon ginger
- ½ teaspoon nutmeg
- ½ teaspoon salt
- 1 pinch clove
- 1 cup 1% low-fat milk
- 6 tablespoons canned pumpkin puree
- 2 tablespoons melted butter
- 1 egg

Directions

1. Whisk flour, sugar, baking powder, spices and salt in a bowl.
2. In a separate bowl whisk together milk, pumpkin, melted butter, and egg.
3. Fold mixture into dry ingredients.
4. Spray or grease a skillet and heat over medium heat: pour in 1/4 cup batter for each pancake.
5. Cook pancakes about 3 minutes per side. Serve with butter and syrup. Makes about six 6-inch pancakes.

Cornflakes with Berries

Ingredients

1. 2 cups cornflakes
2. 1 cup 1% low-fat milk
3. 1 cup berries, fresh or frozen, thawed

Directions

1. Place cornflakes in a small bowl.
2. Top with milk and berries and serve.

Berry Breakfast Quinoa

Ingredients:

- ¼ cup milk
- 2 containers (6 oz each) 99% Fat Free French vanilla, strawberry or peach yogurt
- 4 teaspoons chia seed
- 1 cup cooled cooked quinoa (1/4 cup uncooked)
- 2 cups fresh fruit (mixed berries or chopped peaches)
- ¼ cup coarsely chopped toasted almonds or pecans
- 1/8 teaspoon ground cinnamon

Directions:

1. In medium bowl, stir together milk, yogurt and chia seed until blended. Evenly divide mixture among 4 glasses. Spoon 1/4 cup cooled cooked quinoa on top of yogurt layer on each.
2. Top each with a layer of fruit and almonds. Sprinkle with cinnamon. Let stand 5 minutes, or cover and refrigerate overnight.

Banana-Blueberry Smoothie

Ingredients:

- 1 cup milk
- 1 cup Cheerios cereal
- 1 ripe banana, cut into chunks
- 1 cup fresh blueberries
- 1 cup ice
- Garnishes, If Desired
- Banana slices
- Additional cereal

Directions:

1. In blender, place Smoothie ingredients. Cover; blend on high speed about 30 seconds or until smooth.
2. Pour into 2 glasses. Garnish as desired. Serve immediately.

Cherry Strawberry Smoothie

Ingredients:

- 2 containers (5.3 oz each) honey Greek yogurt
- 1 ½ cups frozen organic cherries
- ½ cup frozen organic strawberries
- 1 cup milk

Directions:

1. In blender, place all ingredients. Cover and blend on high speed about 1 minute or until smooth.
2. Pour into 3 glasses. Serve immediately.

Orange Flaxseed Smoothie

Ingredients

- 2 oranges, cut into segments
- 2 peaches, pitted and sliced
- 1 cup carrot juice
- ¼ teaspoon cinnamon powder
- 1 pinch ground ginger
- 2 tablespoons ground flaxseeds

Directions

1. Combine all the ingredients in a blender. Pulse until smooth and creamy.
2. Serve the smoothie fresh and chilled.

Chapter 5: Salads

Winter Fruit Waldorf Salad

Ingredients:

- 2 medium unpeeled red apples, diced
- 2 medium unpeeled pears, diced
- ½ cup thinly sliced celery
- ½ cup golden raisins
- ½ cup chopped dates
- ¼ cup gluten-free mayonnaise or salad dressing
- ¼ cup 99% Fat Free orange crème yogurt (from 6-oz container)
- 2 tablespoons frozen orange juice concentrate
- 8 cups shredded lettuce
- Walnut halves, if desired

Directions:

1. In large bowl, mix apples, pears, celery, raisins and dates.
2. In small bowl, mix mayonnaise, yogurt and juice concentrate until well blended. Add to fruit; toss to coat. (Salad can be refrigerated up to 1 hour.) Serve on lettuce. Garnish with walnut halves.

Quinoa and Vegetable Salad

Ingredients:

- 1 cup uncooked quinoa
- 2 tablespoons fresh lemon juice
- 2 tablespoons olive oil
- 2 tablespoons chopped fresh basil

- 1 can (15 oz) gluten-free garbanzo beans, drained, rinsed
- 1 can (15.25 oz) gluten-free whole kernel sweet corn, drained
- 1 can (14.5 oz) gluten-free diced tomatoes, drained
- 1 cup chopped red bell pepper
- 1/3 cup quartered pitted olives
- ½ cup crumbled gluten-free feta cheese

Directions:

1. Rinse quinoa under cold water 1 minute; drain. Cook quinoa as directed on package; drain. Cool completely, about 30 minutes.
2. Meanwhile, in small nonmetal bowl, place lemon juice, oil and basil; mix well. Set aside for dressing.
3. In large bowl, gently toss cooked quinoa, beans, corn, tomatoes, bell pepper and olives. Pour dressing over quinoa mixture; toss gently to coat. Serve immediately or refrigerate 1 to 2 hours before serving.

Garden Citrus Salad

Ingredients

- 2 cups baby spinach
- 2 cups arugula leaves
- 1 zucchini, sliced
- 1 red onion, sliced
- 2 tablespoons chopped cilantro
- 1 orange, cut into segments
- 1 lime, juiced
- 2 tablespoons extra virgin olive oil
- Salt and pepper

Directions

1. Combine the baby spinach, arugula leaves, zucchini, red onion, cilantro and orange in a salad bowl.
2. Drizzle in the lime juice and oil then season with salt and pepper. Serve the salad fresh.

Zesty Garden Salad

Ingredients

- 1 teaspoon Dijon mustard
- 1 sprig fresh dill, chopped (optional)
- 1 tablespoon chopped green onion
- 2 tablespoons shredded Cheddar cheese
- ½ cup sweet corn kernels
- ½ cup sugar snap peas
- 1/3 cup frozen shelled edamame (optional)
- 2 cups iceberg lettuce
- 1 pinch salt and pepper

Directions

1. Stir the Dijon mustard, dill, green onion, Cheddar cheese, corn, peas, and edamame in a bowl until evenly combined.
2. Stir in the iceberg lettuce, season to taste with salt and pepper, and toss to mix.

Orange & Duck Confit Salad

Ingredients

- 1 tablespoon sherry vinegar

- 4 blood oranges, divided (3 sectioned, about 1 cup; 1 juiced, about 1/4 cup)
- 1 teaspoon Dijon mustard
- 1 tablespoon olive oil
- ¼ teaspoon salt
- ¼ teaspoon pepper
- 1 small duck confit leg (5-6 ounces), shredded, skin, fat, and bones discarded (about 3/4 cup)
- 6 cups mixed winter salad greens (such as romaine, escarole, and spinach)
- ¼ cup skinned chopped hazelnuts, toasted

Directions

1. In a small bowl, combine vinegar, orange juice, mustard, and oil, whisking well. Whisk in salt and pepper.
2. In a large bowl, combine shredded duck, salad greens, hazelnuts, and orange sections. Drizzle with vinaigrette; serve.

Mom's Potato Salad

Ingredients

- 2 potatoes
- 1 sweet potato
- 4 eggs
- 2 stalks celery, chopped
- ½ onion, chopped
- ¾ cup mayonnaise
- 1 tablespoon prepared mustard
- 1 teaspoon salt
- 1 ½ teaspoons ground black pepper

Directions

1. Bring a large pot of salted water to a boil. Add potatoes and cook until tender but still firm, about 30 minutes. Drain, cool, peel and chop.
2. Place eggs in a saucepan and cover with cold water. Bring water to a boil. Cover, remove from heat, and let eggs stand in hot water for 10 to 12 minutes. Remove from hot water; cool, peel and chop.
3. Combine the potatoes, eggs, celery and onion. Whisk together the mayonnaise, mustard, salt and pepper. Add to potato mixture, toss well to coat. Refrigerate and serve chilled.

Strawberry-Spinach Salad

Ingredients

- 3 cups baby spinach
- 1 cup strawberries, halved
- 1 red onion, sliced
- 1 can of tuna
- 1 tablespoon white wine vinegar
- 1 tablespoon lemon juice
- 1 teaspoon mustard
- 2 tablespoons extra virgin olive oil

Directions

1. Combine the spinach, strawberries, red onion and tuna in a salad bowl.
2. For the dressing, mix the vinegar, lemon juice, mustard and olive oil in a bowl. Add salt and pepper to taste and mix well.
3. Drizzle the dressing over the salad and serve it fresh.

Cherry Tomato Corn Salad

Ingredients

- ¼ cup minced fresh basil
- 3 tablespoons olive oil
- 2 teaspoons lime juice
- 1 teaspoon sugar
- ½ teaspoon salt
- ¼ teaspoon pepper
- 2 cups frozen corn, thawed
- 2 cups cherry tomatoes, halved
- 1 cup chopped seeded and peeled cucumber

Directions

1. In a jar with a tight-fitting lid, combine the basil, oil, lime juice, sugar, salt and pepper; shake well.
2. In a large bowl, combine the corn, tomatoes and cucumber.
3. Drizzle with dressing and toss to coat. Refrigerate until serving.

Summer Watermelon Salad

Ingredients

- ¼ cup balsamic vinegar
- 1 tablespoon Dijon mustard
- 1 tablespoon chopped garlic
- ½ teaspoon salt
- ½ teaspoon freshly ground black pepper
- ¾ cup olive oil
- 3 cups 2-inch cubes watermelon
- 1 cup crumbled feta cheese

- ½ red onion, sliced very thin
- coarsely ground black pepper for taste

Directions

1. Mix the vinegar and Dijon mustard in a bowl. Stir the garlic, salt, and pepper into the mixture. Slowly stream the olive oil into the dressing while whisking vigorously. Place the dressing in the refrigerator until ready to use.
2. Combine the watermelon, feta cheese, and red onion in a large bowl; toss lightly to mix. Season with the coarsely ground black pepper.
3. Pour about half the dressing over the salad; gently toss to coat. Refrigerate the salad at least 30 minutes. Drizzle the remaining dressing over the salad just before serving.

Spinach Grapefruit Salad

Ingredients

- 4 cups baby spinach
- 2 grapefruits, cut into segments
- 1 red onion, sliced
- ¼ cup hazelnuts, chopped
- ½ cup plain yogurt
- 2 tablespoons lemon juice
- 2 tablespoons extra virgin olive oil
- Salt and pepper for taste

Directions

1. Combine the baby spinach, grapefruits, onion and hazelnuts in a bowl.
2. Combine the yogurt, lemon juice, olive oil, salt and pepper in a glass jar.

3. Shake until creamy.
4. Drizzle the dressing over the salad and serve it fresh.

Chunky Vegetable Salad

Ingredients

- 4 tomatoes, cubes
- 1 cup cooked chickpeas, drained
- 1 jalapeno pepper, chopped
- 1 red bell pepper, cored and diced
- 1 celery stalk, sliced
- 1 cucumber, sliced
- 2 tablespoons olive oil
- 1 tablespoon balsamic vinegar
- 1 tablespoon chopped parsley
- 1 tablespoon chopped cilantro
- Add a pinch of salt and pepper.

Directions

1. Combine all the ingredients in a salad bowl.
2. Add salt and pepper and serve the salad warm and fresh.

Chapter 6: Soups & Appetizers

Roasted Garlic & Cauliflower Soup

Ingredients

- 1 large head cauliflower (about 2 ½ lb.)
- 4 ½ teaspoons olive oil
- 1 ½ teaspoons kosher salt
- 3 garlic cloves, divided & unpeeled
- 3 cups chicken broth
- 1 cup 2% reduced-fat milk
- ½ cup grated Parmesan cheese
- Freshly ground black pepper
- Garnishes: olive oil, pomegranate seeds, fresh thyme leaves

Directions

1. Preheat oven to 425 °. Cut cauliflower into 2-inch florets; toss with olive oil and 1/ 2 tsp. salt. Arrange florets in a single layer on a jelly-roll pan. Wrap garlic cloves in aluminum foil, and place on jelly-roll pan with cauliflower.
2. Bake at 425 ° for 30 to 40 minutes or until cauliflower is golden brown, tossing cauliflower every 15 minutes.
3. Transfer cauliflower to a large Dutch oven. Unwrap garlic, and cool 5 minutes. Peel garlic, and add to cauliflower. Add stock, and bring to a simmer over medium heat; simmer, stirring occasionally, 5 minutes. Let mixture cool 10 minutes.
4. Process cauliflower mixture, in batches, in a blender until smooth, stopping to scrape down sides as needed.
5. Return cauliflower mixture to Dutch oven; stir in milk, cheese, and remaining 1 tsp. salt. Cook over low heat,

stirring occasionally, 2 to 3 minutes or until thoroughly heated. Add pepper for taste.

Lentil Soup

Ingredients:

- 1 cup regular lentils
- ¼ cup wild rice
- ¼ cup barley,
- 4 cups vegetable broth
- 2 cups chopped kale
- sea salt, pepper

Directions:

1. In a large pot, add the broth and let it boil.
2. Add the rest of the ingredients and seasoning.
3. Cover and let it simmer for about 40 min.
4. Add the kale and let it cook for about 15 more min.

Carrot Soup

Ingredients:

- 2 bags (1 lb each) ready-to-eat baby-cut carrots
- 2 large onions, chopped (about 2 cups)
- 5 ¼ cups chicken broth (from two 32-oz cartons)
- ½ teaspoon salt
- ½ cup whipping cream
- ½ cup orange juice
- 3 tablespoons packed brown sugar
- 2 tablespoons grated gingerroot
- ¼ teaspoon white pepper

- Fresh orange slices, quartered, if desired
- Fresh Italian parsley, if desired

Directions:

1. Spray 4- to 5-quart slow cooker with cooking spray. In cooker, mix carrots, onions, broth and salt.
2. Cover; cook on Low heat setting 8 to 10 hours.
3. Pour 4 cups of the soup mixture to blender; add half each of the whipping cream, orange juice, brown sugar, gingerroot and pepper. Cover and blend until smooth; return to cooker. Blend remaining soup mixture with remaining half of ingredients; return to cooker.
4. Increase heat setting to High. Cover; cook 15 to 20 minutes longer or until hot. Garnish individual servings with an orange quarter and parsley.

Home-Style Potato Soup

Ingredients

- 3 medium potatoes (about 1 pound)
- 1 ¾ cups chicken broth (from 32-ounce carton)
- 2 medium green onions with tops
- 1 ½ cups milk
- ¼ teaspoon salt
- 1/8 teaspoon pepper
- 1/8 teaspoon dried thyme leaves

Directions

1. Peel the potatoes, and cut into large pieces.
2. Heat the chicken broth and potatoes to boiling in the saucepan over high heat, stirring occasionally with a fork to make sure potatoes do not stick to the saucepan. Once mixture is boiling, reduce heat just enough so mixture

bubbles gently. Cover and cook about 15 minutes or until potatoes are tender when pierced with a fork.
3. While the potatoes are cooking, peel and thinly slice the green onions. If you have extra onions, wrap them airtight and store in the refrigerator up to 5 days.
4. When the potatoes are done, remove the saucepan from the heat, but do not drain. Break the potatoes into smaller pieces with the potato masher or large fork. The mixture should still be lumpy.
5. Stir the milk, salt, pepper, thyme and onions into the potato mixture. Heat over medium heat, stirring occasionally, until hot and steaming, but do not let the soup boil.

Greek Cold Cucumber Soup

Ingredients

- 4 cucumbers
- 2 cups plain yogurt
- 2 garlic cloves
- Salt and pepper
- 2 tablespoons lemon juice
- 2 tablespoons chopped dill

Directions

1. Combine the cucumbers, yogurt, garlic, lemon juice, salt and pepper in a blender.
2. Pulse until smooth.
3. Stir in the dill and serve the soup chilled.

Gazpacho

Ingredients

- 1 hothouse cucumber. halved and seeded, but not peeled
- 2 red bell peppers, cored and seeded
- 4 plum tomatoes
- 1 red onion
- 2 garlic cloves, minced
- 3 cups tomato juice
- ¼ cup white wine vinegar
- ¼ cup olive oil
- ½ tablespoon salt
- 1 teaspoon freshly ground black pepper

Directions

1. Roughly chop the cucumbers, bell peppers, tomatoes, and red onions into 1-inch cubes.
2. Put each vegetable separately into a food processor fitted with a steel blade and pulse until it is coarsely chopped.
3. Once each vegetable is processed, combine them in a large bowl and add the garlic, tomato juice, vinegar, olive oil, salt, and pepper. Mix well and chill before serving.

Mint Ginger Sweet Potato Soup

Ingredients

- 1 tablespoon olive oil
- 2 medium-large sweet potatoes peeled, chopped, and pureed
- 1 clove garlic
- 1 teaspoon ginger

- 1/3 teaspoon turmeric
- 4 diced mint leaves
- 2 cups vegetable broth

Directions

1. Pour olive oil into food processor.
2. Add the washed, peeled and pieces of sweet potato into the food processor with the oil.
3. Add garlic clove to the food processor.
4. Add the ginger turmeric.
5. Wash, dry, and chop mint leaves.
6. Puree.
7. Pour into medium sized pot or Dutch oven.
8. Add broth.
9. Let sit over medium heat for 25-30 minutes.

Creamy Garlic Zucchini Soup

Ingredients

- 2 tablespoons extra virgin olive oil
- 4 garlic cloves, chopped
- 1 shallot, chopped
- 3 zucchinis, cubed
- 2 potatoes, peeled and cubed
- 2 cups water
- 2 cups vegetable stock
- Salt and pepper to taste

Directions:

1. Heat the oil in a soup pot and add the garlic and shallot.
2. Cook for a few seconds then add the rest of the ingredients.

3. Season with salt and pepper and cook on low heat for 15 minutes.
4. When done, puree the soup with an immersion blender.
5. Pour the soup into serving bowls

Vegetables & Hummus

Ingredients

- ¾ cup mixed vegetables, such as baby carrots, cherry tomatoes and red bell pepper slices
- 1 (15.5 ounce) can garbanzo beans (chickpeas), drained 1/3 cup pitted Spanish Manzanilla olives
- 1 teaspoon minced garlic
- 3 tablespoons olive oil
- 2 tablespoons lemon juice
- 1 ½ teaspoons chopped fresh basil
- 1 teaspoon cilantro leaves
- salt and pepper for taste

Directions

1. Wash vegetables and a slice them into bitable sizes.
2. Place garbanzo beans, olives, and garlic into the bowl of a blender or food processor. Pour in olive oil and lemon juice; season with basil, cilantro, salt, and pepper.
3. Cover and puree until smooth.
4. Arrange vegetables on a platter.
5. Dip into hummus and eat.

Deviled Eggs

Ingredients

- 12 eggs 1 jalapeno pepper, minced
- 1 habanero peppers, seeded and minced
- ¼ cup mayonnaise
- 1 teaspoon yellow mustard
- 1/8 teaspoon paprika

Directions

1. Place the eggs into a saucepan in a single layer, and fill with water to cover the eggs by at least 1 inch. Bring the water to a boil over high heat. Cover, and remove from the heat; let the eggs stand in the hot water for 15 minutes. Pour out the hot water, then cool the eggs under cold running water in the sink. Peel.
2. Cut the cooled eggs in half lengthwise. Remove the yolks, and place them into a mixing bowl along with the jalapeno, habanero, mayonnaise, and mustard; mash together until smooth. Transfer the yolk mixture to a pastry bag, and decoratively squeeze into the white halves. Sprinkle with paprika to garnish.

Zucchini Boats

Ingredients

- 2 zucchinis
- 1 pound ground chicken
- 1 teaspoon dried basil
- 1 teaspoon dried oregano
- 2 tablespoons chopped parsley
- 1 shallot, chopped
- Salt and pepper for taste

- 1 cup tomato sauce
- ½ cup dry white wine
- 1 bay leaf

Directions

1. Cut the zucchinis in half and carefully scoop out the flesh. Chop the zucchini flesh finely and place it in a bowl.
2. Add the ground chicken, basil, oregano, parsley and shallot and season with salt and pepper. Spoon the mixture back into the zucchini boats.
3. Place the zucchini in a deep dish baking tray and pour in the tomato sauce and wine.
4. Add the bay leaf and a pinch of salt and pepper.
5. Cook in the preheated oven at 350F for 15-20 minutes.
6. Serve the zucchini boats warm.

Caprese Appetizer

Ingredients

- 20 grape tomatoes
- 10 ounces mozzarella cheese, cubed
- 2 tablespoons extra virgin olive oil
- 2 tablespoons fresh basil leaves, chopped
- 1 pinch salt
- 1 pinch ground black pepper
- 20 toothpicks

Directions

1. Toss tomatoes, mozzarella cheese, olive oil, basil, salt, and pepper together in a bowl until well coated.
2. Skewer one tomato and one piece of mozzarella cheese on each toothpick.

Kale & Tofu

Ingredients

- 3 oz. fresh kale leaves
- 3 oz. firm tofu cubes
- Olive oil for drizzling
- No-salt seasoning

Directions

1. Prepare baking tray and preheat oven to 400.
2. Layout individual kale leaves, drop one tofu cube in the center. Fold leaf ends over tofu cube and flip.
3. Drizzle with olive oil and seasoning Bake 18-22 minutes.

Minestrone Soup

Ingredients

- 2 tablespoons extra virgin olive oil
- 1 shallot, chopped 1 red bell pepper, cored and diced
- 2 carrots, diced
- 1 parsnip, diced
- 1 celery stalk, sliced
- 1 zucchini, cubed
- 2 cups green beans, chopped
- ½ cup green peas
- 2 cups baby spinach
- 1 cup diced tomatoes
- 4 cups water
- 2 cups vegetable stock
- ½ teaspoon dried oregano

- ½ teaspoon dried basil
- Salt and pepper to taste

Directions

1. Combine the olive oil and the vegetables in a soup pot.
2. Add the water, stock and herbs, as well as salt and pepper and cook on medium heat for 20-25 minutes.
3. Serve the soup warm and fresh, although it tastes just as good chilled.

Chapter 7: Chicken

Asparagus Chicken Divan

Ingredients

- 1 pound skinless, boneless
- chicken breast halves
- 2 pounds fresh asparagus, trimmed
- 1 (10.75 ounce) can condensed cream of chicken soup, undiluted
- 1 teaspoon Worcestershire sauce
- ¼ teaspoon ground nutmeg
- 1 cup grated Parmesan cheese,
- ½ cup whipping cream, whipped
- ¾ cup mayonnaise*

Directions

1. Broil chicken 6 in. from the heat until juices run clear.
2. Meanwhile, in a large skillet, bring 1/2 in. of water to a boil. Add asparagus. Reduce heat; cover and simmer for 3-5 minutes or until crisp and tender.
3. Drain and place in a greased shallow 2-1/2-qt. baking dish.
4. Cut chicken into thin slices. In a bowl, combine the soup, Worcestershire sauce and nutmeg. Spread half over asparagus. Sprinkle with 1/3 cup Parmesan cheese. Top with chicken. Spread remaining soup mixture over chicken; sprinkle with 1/3 cup Parmesan cheese.
5. Bake, uncovered, at 400 degrees F for 20 minutes. Fold whipped cream into mayonnaise; spread over top. Sprinkle with remaining Parmesan cheese. Broil 4-6 in. from the heat for about 2 minutes or until golden brown.

Balsamic Chicken Breasts

Ingredients

- 2 sweet potatoes, peeled and cut into 2-inch pieces
- 1 tablespoon olive oil
- 2 skinless, boneless chicken breast halves
- ½ cup balsamic vinegar salt and ground black pepper for taste
- ½ cup balsamic vinegar

Directions

1. Preheat oven to 400 degrees F (200 degrees C).
2. Place the potatoes on a baking sheet; drizzle olive oil over potatoes and season with salt and pepper.
3. Place the chicken breasts in a baking dish. Pour 1/2 cup of balsamic vinegar over the breasts; season with salt and pepper. Cover with aluminum foil. Place the potatoes in the preheated oven and bake for 10 minutes; place the dish with the chicken in the oven and cook both the potatoes and chicken another 20 minutes; flip both the potatoes and chicken; reduce the oven heat to 350 degrees F (175 degrees C).
4. Bake another 20 minutes.
5. Pour ½ cup of balsamic vinegar into a small saucepan and place over medium heat. Cook until reduced to about ¼ cup. Place the chicken breasts atop the potatoes; drizzle with the reduced balsamic vinegar to serve.

Caribbean-Spiced Roast Chicken

Ingredients

- 1 ½ tablespoons fresh lime juice
- 2 fluid ounces rum
- 1 tablespoon brown sugar
- ¼ teaspoon cayenne pepper
- ¼ teaspoon ground clove
- ½ teaspoon ground cinnamon
- ½ teaspoon ground ginger
- 1 teaspoon black pepper
- ½ teaspoon salt
- ½ teaspoon dried thyme leaves
- 1 (3 pound) whole chicken
- 1 tablespoon vegetable oil

Directions

1. Preheat oven to 325 degrees F (165 degrees C).
2. In a small bowl, combine the lime juice, rum, and brown sugar; set aside. Mix together the cayenne pepper, clove, cinnamon, ginger, pepper, salt, and thyme leaves. Brush the chicken with oil, then coat with the spice mixture.
3. Place in a roasting pan, and bake about 90 minutes, until the juices run clear or until a meat thermometer inserted in thickest part of the thigh reaches 180 degrees F. Baste the chicken with the sauce every 20 minutes while it's cooking. Allow chicken to rest for 10 minutes before carving.

Sage and Garlic Grilled Chicken Breasts

Ingredients:

- 1 teaspoon dried sage leaves
- ½ teaspoon seasoned salt
- ½ teaspoon dried marjoram leaves
- ¼ teaspoon coarse ground black pepper
- 2 garlic cloves, minced
- 2 tablespoons olive oil
- 4 boneless skinless chicken breast halves

Directions:

1. Heat closed contact grill for 5 minutes.
2. Meanwhile, in small bowl, combine all ingredients except chicken breast halves; mix well. Place chicken on sheet of waxed paper. Brush or rub mixture onto all sides of chicken.
3. When grill is heated, place chicken on bottom grill surface. Close grill; cook 5 to 7 minutes or until chicken is fork-tender and juices run clear.

Herb & Garlic Chicken with Vegetables

Ingredients:

- 1 cut-up whole chicken (3 to 3 1/2 lb)
- 2 tablespoons olive or vegetable oil
- 1 envelope savory herb with garlic soup mix (from 2.4-oz box)
- 1/3 cup chicken broth
- 4 medium stalks celery, cut in half lengthwise, then cut into 4-inch pieces
- 1 large onion, cut into 6 wedges
- 2 large carrots, cut in half lengthwise, then cut into 4-inch pieces
- 2 medium unpeeled russet potatoes, each cut into 8 pieces

Directions:

1. Heat oven to 425°F. Remove skin from chicken if desired. In small bowl, mix oil, soup mix and broth. Brush both sides of chicken pieces with about half of the oil mixture.
2. In large bowl, mix celery, onion, carrots, potatoes and remaining oil mixture. Arrange vegetables in ungreased 15x10x1-inch pan. Bake 15 minutes.
3. Place chicken pieces in pan, overlapping vegetables if necessary. Bake 35 to 40 minutes longer or until vegetables are tender and juice of chicken is clear when thickest piece is cut to bone (170°F for breasts; 180°F for thighs and legs).

Chicken Cacciatore

Ingredients

- 6 chicken thighs
- 2 tablespoons extra virgin olive
- oil 1 sweet onion, chopped 2 garlic cloves, minced
- 2 red bell peppers, cored and diced
- 2 carrots, diced
- 1 rosemary sprig
- 1 thyme sprig
- 4 tomatoes, peeled and diced
- ½ cup tomato juice
- ¼ cup dry white wine
- 1 cup chicken stock
- Salt and pepper to taste
- 1 bay leaf

Directions

1. Heat the oil in a heavy saucepan.
2. Add the chicken and cook on all sides until golden.
3. Stir in the onion and garlic and cook for 2 minutes.
4. Stir in the rest of the ingredients and season with salt and pepper.
5. Cook on low heat for 30 minutes.
6. Serve the chicken cacciatore warm.

Chicken Marsala

Ingredients

- 4 chicken fillets
- 1 tablespoon cornstarch
- 2 tablespoons extra virgin olive oil
- 2 prosciutto slices, chopped
- 1 pound button mushrooms
- ¼ cup Marsala wine
- 1 cup chicken stock
- Salt and pepper to taste

Directions

1. Season the chicken with salt and pepper then sprinkle with cornstarch.
2. Heat the oil in a saucepan and place the chicken in the hot oil.
3. Cook on each side until golden then add the rest of the ingredients.
4. Season with salt and pepper and cook on low heat for 25 minutes.
5. Serve the chicken and the sauce warm.

Braised Chicken with Wild Mushrooms and Thyme

Ingredients

- 1 cup boiling water
- ½ oz dried porcini mushrooms
- 1 tablespoon butter
- 1 tablespoon olive oil
- 1 cut-up broiler-fryer chicken (3 to 3 1/2 lb)
- 2 large onions, chopped (2 cups)
- 5 cloves garlic, finely chopped
- 6 medium button mushrooms, sliced
- 2 medium carrots, chopped (1 cup)
- 2 medium stalks celery, chopped (1 cup)
- 2 dried bay leaves
- 2 fresh thyme sprigs or 1 teaspoon dried thyme leaves
- 5 tablespoons chopped fresh parsley
- 1 cup chicken broth
- ½ cup dry white wine or chicken broth
- 1 can (14.5 oz) diced tomatoes, undrained
- ¼ teaspoon salt
- ¼ teaspoon freshly ground pepper

Directions

1. Adjust oven rack to middle position. Heat oven to 300°F.
2. In small bowl, pour boiling water over dried mushrooms. Let stand 30 minutes to allow mushrooms to rehydrate (if mushrooms float to surface, place small saucer in bowl to keep them submerged). Use slotted spoon to remove rehydrated mushrooms from water; set aside. Reserve mushroom water.

3. In 4- or 5-quart ovenproof Dutch oven, heat butter and oil over medium-high heat until butter is melted. Add half of the chicken pieces and cook 6 minutes, turning occasionally, until chicken is deep golden brown (you are not cooking the chicken, just giving it color). Remove chicken from Dutch oven and place on plate. Repeat with remaining chicken.
4. Reduce heat to medium and add onions and garlic. Cook 5 minutes, stirring occasionally, until soft. Add rehydrated and sliced button mushrooms, carrots, celery, bay leaves, thyme and 3 tablespoons of the parsley. Cook 5 minutes, stirring occasionally, until vegetables are softened and mushrooms give up their juices.
5. Add reserved mushroom water and heat to a simmer. Simmer uncovered 10 minutes (you are trying to concentrate the flavor of the liquid). Add chicken (along with any juices that may have accumulated on plate), broth, wine, tomatoes, salt and pepper.
6. Cover pan and place in oven. Bake 1 1/2 hours or until chicken is very tender and there is a good amount of broth. Remove and discard bay leaves and thyme sprig. Place 2 pieces chicken into each of 4 large, flat serving bowls and ladle broth over. Sprinkle with remaining 2 tablespoons parsley.

Chapter 8: Turkey

Grilled Turkey Tenderloins

Ingredients

- ¼ cup reduced-sodium soy sauce
- 4 teaspoons canola oil
- 1 teaspoon sugar
- 1 garlic clove, minced
- ½ teaspoon ground ginger
- ½ teaspoon ground mustard
- ¾ pound turkey breast tenderloins

Directions

1. In a bowl, combine the soy sauce, oil, sugar, garlic, ginger and mustard. Pour 1/4 cup marinade into a large resealable plastic bag; add the turkey. Seal bag and turn to coat; refrigerate for up to 4 hours. Cover and refrigerate remaining marinade for basting.
2. Coat grill rack with nonstick cooking spray before starting the grill. Drain and discard marinade from turkey. Grill turkey, covered, over medium heat for 8-10 minutes or until a meat thermometer reads 170 degrees F, turning twice and basting occasionally with reserved marinade. Cut into slices.

Mom's Turkey Meatloaf

Ingredients

- 1 ½ pounds ground turkey
- 1 small onion, minced

- 2 stalks celery, minced
- 3 cloves garlic, minced
- 2 teaspoons chopped fresh basil
- ¼ cup Parmesan cheese
- ½ cup whole wheat bread crumbs
- 1 egg
- ¼ cup milk
- 1 (10.75 ounce) can condensed tomato soup

Directions

1. Preheat an oven to 350 degrees F (175 degrees C). Prepare a 9x13 inch baking dish with cooking spray.
2. Mix the ground turkey, onion, celery, garlic, basil, Parmesan cheese, bread crumbs, egg, and milk together in a large bowl. Shape the mixture into a loaf and place into prepared pan. Pour the tomato soup over the meatloaf. Cover tightly with aluminum foil.
3. Bake in the preheated oven until no longer pink in the center, about 45 minutes. An instant-read thermometer inserted into the center should read at least 165 degrees F (74 degrees C).

Turkey Spinach Patties

Ingredients:

- 1 pound ground turkey
- 1 cup baby spinach, chopped
- 4 garlic cloves, minced
- ½ teaspoon dried basil
- 1 shallot, chopped
- 1 egg yolk
- Salt and pepper for taste

Directions

1. Mix the turkey with the spinach, garlic, basil, shallot and egg yolk in a bowl. Add salt and pepper to taste and mix well.
2. Form 6 patties and place them aside.
3. Heat a grill pan over medium flame and place the patties on the grill.
4. Cook on each side for 4-5 minutes until browned.
5. Serve the turkey patties warm.

Grilled Turkey Kabobs

Ingredients

- 1/3 cup chili sauce
- 2 tablespoons lemon juice
- 1 tablespoon sugar
- 2 bay leaves
- 1 pound turkey breast tenderloins, cut into 1/2-inch cubes
- 2 medium zucchini, cut into 1/2 inch slices
- 2 small green peppers, cut into 1 1/2 inch squares
- 2 small onions, quartered
- 8 medium fresh mushrooms
- 8 cherry tomatoes
- 1 tablespoon canola oil

Directions

1. In a bowl, combine the chili sauce, lemon juice, sugar and bay leaves; mix well. Pour 1/4 cup marinade into a large resealable plastic bag; add the turkey. Seal bag and turn to coat; refrigerate for at least 2 hours or overnight. Cover and refrigerate remaining marinade.

2. Coat grill rack with nonstick cooking spray before starting the grill. Drain and discard marinade. Discard bay leaves from reserved marinade. On eight metal or soaked wooden skewers, alternately thread turkey and vegetables. Brush lightly with oil.
3. Grill, uncovered, over medium-hot heat for 3-4 minutes on each side or until juices run clear, basting frequently with reserved marinade and turning three times.

Spiced Turkey Patties in Tomato Sauce

Ingredients

- 1 can diced tomatoes
- 1 ½ cups chicken stock
- 1 bay leaf
- 2 tablespoons tomato paste
- 2 pounds ground turkey
- 1 carrot, grated
- ½ teaspoon chili powder
- ½ teaspoon cumin powder
- ½ teaspoon dried oregano
- 1 red onion, chopped
- 6 garlic cloves, minced
- 1 teaspoon ground coriander
- Salt and pepper to taste

Directions

1. Combine the tomatoes, stock, bay leaf and tomato paste in a deep dish baking pan.
2. For the patties, mix the turkey, carrot, spices, onion and garlic in a bowl. Add salt and pepper to taste and mix well. Form small patties and place them in the tomato sauce.

3. Cover with aluminum foil and cook in the preheated oven at 350F for 35 minutes.
4. Serve the patties and sauce warm.

Caprese Turkey Burger

Ingredients

- 1 tablespoon balsamic vinegar
- 1 tablespoon extra virgin olive oil
- 4 thick slices tomato
- 1 1/3 pounds lean ground turkey
- 1 tablespoon tomato paste
- ¼ cup chopped fresh basil
- ¼ cup grated Parmesan cheese
- 1 clove garlic, minced
- ¼ teaspoon black pepper
- 4 ounces fresh mozzarella cheese, sliced
- 4 hamburger buns, split

Directions

1. Whisk the balsamic vinegar, oil, salt, and pepper in a small bowl. Pour over tomato slices to marinate.
2. Preheat an outdoor grill for medium-high heat, and lightly oil the grate.
3. Mix ground turkey, tomato paste, basil, Parmesan cheese, garlic, and 1I4 teaspoon pepper in a large bowl. Form beef mixture into 4 equal patties.
4. Cook on the preheated grill until the burgers are cooked to your desired degree of doneness, about 5 minutes per side for well done. An instant-read thermometer inserted into the center should read 160 degrees F (70

degrees C). Top each turkey burger with mozzarella cheese; allow to melt. Serve on hamburger buns with marinated tomato slices

Goat Cheese and Spinach Turkey Burgers

- 1 ½ pounds ground turkey breast
- 1 cup frozen chopped spinach, thawed and drained
- 2 tablespoons goat cheese, crumbled
- 4 hamburger buns, split

Directions

1. Preheat the oven broiler.
2. In a medium bowl, mix ground turkey, spinach, and goat cheese. Form the mixture into 4 patties.
3. Arrange patties on a broiler pan, and place in the center of the preheated oven 15 minutes, or until done.

Spicy Turkey Burgers

Ingredients

- 2 pounds lean ground turkey
- 2 tablespoons minced garlic
- 1 teaspoon minced fresh ginger root
- 2 fresh green chile peppers, diced
- 1 medium red onion, diced
- ½ cup fresh cilantro, finely chopped
- 1 teaspoon salt
- ¼ cup low sodium soy sauce
- 1 tablespoon freshly ground black pepper
- 3 tablespoons paprika
- 1 tablespoon ground dry mustard

- 1 tablespoon ground cumin
- 1 dash Worcestershire sauce
- 4 hamburger buns, split

Directions

1. Preheat the grill for high heat.
2. In a bowl, mix the ground turkey, garlic, ginger, chile peppers, red onion, cilantro, salt, soy sauce, black pepper, paprika, mustard, cumin, and Worcestershire sauce. Form the mixture into 8 burger patties. Lightly oil the grill grate.
3. Place turkey burgers on the grill, and cook 5 to 10 minutes per side, until well done.

Chapter 9: Fish

Roasted Sea Bass

Ingredients

- 6 sea bass fillets
- 1 chili, chopped
- ½ teaspoon cumin powder
- 2 tablespoons extra virgin olive oil
- 2 tablespoons lemon juice
- 1 rosemary sprig
- 1 pound potatoes, peeled
- Salt and pepper to taste

Directions

1. Season the sea bass with salt and pepper.
2. Combine the chili, cumin powder, oil, lemon juice, rosemary sprig and potatoes in a deep dish baking pan.
3. Place the sea bass on top and seal the pan with aluminum foil.
4. Cook in the preheated oven at 350F for 30 minutes. Serve the dish warm.

Roasted Salmon and Vegetables

Ingredients:

- 4 salmon steaks, ½ inch thick (about 1 ½ lb)
- 2 cups refrigerated new potato wedges with skins (from 20-oz bag)
- 2 small zucchini, quartered lengthwise, then cut into 2-inch pieces
- 1 medium red bell pepper, cut into 2-inch pieces

- 1 tablespoon lemon juice
- 1 tablespoon butter or margarine, melted
- ½ teaspoon salt
- ¼ to ½ teaspoon dried tarragon leaves
- ¼ teaspoon pepper

Directions:

1. Heat oven to 425°F. Place salmon steaks in ungreased 15x10x1-inch pan. Arrange potato wedges, zucchini and bell pepper around salmon.
2. Brush salmon with lemon juice. Brush salmon and vegetables with butter; sprinkle with salt, tarragon and pepper.
3. Bake 25 to 35 minutes or until salmon flakes easily with fork and vegetables are tender.

Grilled Tuna Steaks

Ingredients

- 8 (3 ounce) fillets fresh tuna steaks, 1 inch thick
- ½ cup soy sauce
- 1/3 cup sherry
- ¼ cup Olive oil
- 1 tablespoon fresh lime juice
- 1 clove garlic, minced

Directions

1. Place tuna steaks in a shallow baking dish. In a medium bowl, mix soy sauce, sherry, olive oil, fresh lime juice, and garlic. Pour the soy sauce mixture over the tuna steaks, and turn to coat. Cover, and refrigerate for at least one hour.
2. Preheat grill for high heat. Lightly oil grill grate.

3. Place tuna steaks on grill, and discard remaining marinade. Grill for 3 to 6 minutes per side, or to your preference.

Grilled Lemon Garlic Halibut Steaks

Ingredients

- ¼ cup lemon juice
- 1 tablespoon vegetable oil
- ¼ teaspoon salt
- ¼ teaspoon pepper
- 2 cloves garlic, finely chopped
- 4 halibut or tuna steaks, about 1 inch thick (about 2 pounds)
- ¼ cup chopped fresh parsley
- 1 tablespoon grated lemon peel

Directions

1. Brush grill rack with vegetable oil. Heat coals or gas grill for direct heat. In shallow glass or plastic dish or resealable food-storage plastic bag, mix lemon juice, 1 tablespoon oil, the salt, pepper and garlic. Add fish; turn several times to coat with marinade. Cover dish or seal bag and refrigerate 10 minutes.
2. Remove fish from marinade; reserve marinade. Cover and grill fish 4 to 6 inches from medium heat 10 to 15 minutes, turning once and brushing with marinade, until fish flakes easily with fork. Discard any remaining marinade.
3. Sprinkle fish with parsley and lemon peel.

Lemony Halibut

Instructions

- 6 (6 ounce) fillets halibut
- 3 teaspoons dried dill weed
- 3 teaspoons onion powder
- ¼ teaspoon paprika seasoning
- salt to taste
- 1pinch lemon pepper
- 2 teaspoons dried parsley
- 1 pinch garlic powder
- 2 tablespoons lemon juice

Directions

1. Preheat oven to 375 degrees F (190 degrees C). Cut 6 foil squares, large enough for the size of each fillet. Center fillets on the foil squares and sprinkle each with dill weed, onion powder, paprika, seasoned salt, lemon pepper, parsley and garlic powder.
2. Sprinkle lemon juice over each fillet. Fold foil over fillets to make a pocket. Pleat seams to securely enclose.
3. Place packets on a baking sheet and bake in the preheat oven for 30 minutes.

Green Salmon Burgers

Ingredients

- 4 salmon fillets
- 4 garlic cloves, minced
- 2 tablespoons chopped dill
- 1 tablespoon chopped parsley
- 4 garlic cloves, minced

- 1 tablespoon green curry paste
- Salt and pepper

Directions

1. Place the salmon in a food processor and pulse until well mixed and ground.
2. Add the rest of the ingredients and season with salt and pepper.
3. Form 4 burgers.
4. Heat a grill pan over medium flame. Place the burgers on the grill and cook for 3-4 minutes on each side.
5. Serve the burgers warm with your favorite toppings.

Tilapia Fish Tacos

Ingredients

- 1 cup of corn
- ½ cup diced red onion
- 1 cup peeled, chopped jicama
- ½ cup diced red bell pepper
- 1 cup fresh cilantro leaves
- finely chopped 1 lime, zested and juiced
- 2 tablespoons sour cream
- 2 tablespoons cayenne pepper
- 1 tablespoon ground black pepper
- 2 tablespoons salt
- 6 (4 ounce) fillets tilapia
- 2 tablespoons olive oil
- 12 corn tortillas, warmed

Directions

1. Preheat grill for high heat. In a medium bowl, mix together corn, red onion, jicama, red bell pepper, and cilantro. Stir in lime juice and zest.
2. In a small bowl, combine cayenne pepper, ground black pepper, and salt.
3. Brush each fillet with olive oil, and sprinkle with spices.
4. Arrange fillets on grill grate, and cook for 3 minutes per side. For each fiery fish taco, top two corn tortillas with fish, sour cream, and corn salsa.

Asian Poached Sea Bass

Ingredients

- 4 sea bass fillets
- 1 teaspoon grated ginger
- 2 garlic cloves, sliced
- 1 tablespoon soy sauce
- 1 teaspoon black peppercorns
- 1 teaspoon sesame oil
- 2 cups vegetable stock

Directions

1. Combine the ginger, garlic, soy sauce, peppercorns and sesame oil in a pot, then add the stock also well and bring to a boil.
2. Place the fish in the pot and cover with a lid.
3. Cook for 7-8 minutes then carefully remove the fish and serve.

Rainbow Trout Cooked in Foil

Ingredients

- 2 rainbow trout fillets
- 1 tablespoon olive oil
- 2 teaspoons garlic salt
- 1 teaspoon ground black pepper
- 1 fresh jalapeno pepper
- 1 lemon, sliced

Directions

1. Preheat oven to 400 degrees F (200 degrees C). Rinse fish, and pat dry. Rub fillets with olive oil, and season with garlic salt and black pepper.
2. Place each fillet on a large sheet of aluminum foil. Top with jalapeno slices, and squeeze the juice from the ends of the lemons over the fish. Arrange lemon slices on top of fillets. Carefully seal all edges of the foil to form enclosed packets. Place packets on baking sheet.
3. Bake in preheated oven for 15 to 20 minutes, depending on the size of fish. Fish is done when it flakes easily with a fork.

Chapter 10: Meatless

Lasagna Primavera

Ingredients

- 12 uncooked lasagna noodles
- 3 cups frozen broccoli cuts, thawed and well drained
- 3 large carrots, coarsely shredded (2 cups)
- 2 cups organic diced tomatoes (from 28-oz can), well drained
- 2 medium bell peppers, cut into 1/2-inch pieces
- 1 container (15 oz) ricotta cheese
- ½ cup grated Parmesan cheese
- 1 egg
- 2 containers (10 oz each) refrigerated Alfredo pasta sauce
- 1 package (16 oz) shredded mozzarella cheese (4 cups)

Directions

1. Heat oven to 350°F. Cook and drain noodles as directed on package.
2. Meanwhile, if necessary, cut broccoli florets into bite-size pieces. In large bowl, mix broccoli, carrots, tomatoes and bell peppers. In small bowl, mix ricotta cheese, Parmesan cheese and egg.
3. In ungreased 13x9-inch (3-quart) glass baking dish, spread 2/3 cup Alfredo sauce. Top with 4 noodles. Spread half of the cheese mixture and 2 1/2 cups of the vegetables over noodles. Spoon 2/3 cup sauce in dollops over vegetables. Sprinkle with 1 cup of the mozzarella cheese.
4. Top with 4 noodles; spread with remaining cheese mixture and 2 1/2 cups of vegetables. Spoon 2/3 cup

sauce in dollops over vegetables. Sprinkle with 1 cup mozzarella cheese. Top with remaining 4 noodles and the vegetables. Spoon remaining
sauce in dollops over vegetables. Sprinkle with remaining 2 cups mozzarella cheese.
5. Bake uncovered 45 to 60 minutes or until bubbly and hot in center. Let stand 15 minutes before cutting.

Zucchini Spaghetti

Ingredients:

- 6 oz. uncooked spaghetti
- 3 cups chopped zucchini (2 medium)
- 1/3 cup water
- 1 tablespoon tomato paste
- ¼ teaspoon kosher (coarse) salt
- 1/8 teaspoon coarse ground black pepper
- 1 can (15.5 oz) great northern beans, drained, rinsed
- 1 can (14.5 oz) diced tomatoes with basil, garlic and oregano, undrained
- ½ cup crumbled feta cheese (2 oz)

Directions:

1. Cook spaghetti as directed on package, omitting salt and oil; drain.
2. Meanwhile, spray 12-inch skillet with olive oil cooking spray; heat over medium-high heat. Add zucchini; cook 5 minutes, stirring occasionally, until lightly browned. Stir in water, tomato paste, salt, pepper, beans and tomatoes. Cover; simmer 4 minutes or until thoroughly heated.
3. On each of 4 plates, place about 2/3 cup spaghetti. Top each with 1 cup zucchini mixture and 2 tablespoons cheese.

Walnut Parsley Pesto Spaghetti

Ingredients

- 8 oz whole wheat spaghetti
- ½ cup walnuts
- 1 ½ cups parsley
- 3 garlic cloves
- 2 tablespoons lemon juice
- 4 tablespoons extra virgin olive oil
- Salt and pepper for taste

Directions

1. Pour a few cups of water in a large pot. Add salt and bring to a boil.
2. Throw in the spaghetti and cook for 8 minutes until al dente. Drain well.
3. For the pesto, combine the walnuts, parsley, garlic, lemon juice and olive oil.
4. Add salt and pepper to taste and pulse until the pesto is creamy and smooth.
5. Mix the pesto with cooked spaghetti and serve.

Mac & Cheese

Ingredients

- 1 tablespoon vegetable oil
- 1 tablespoon butter
- 1 teaspoon garlic and parsley powder
- 1 teaspoon onion powder
- 1 tablespoon sriracha sauce
- 1 cup low or no sodium chicken bouillon

- ½ cup low fat milk
- 18 oz. box elbow macaroni
- 1 cup Monterey Jack cheese
- ½ cups plain bread crumbs

Directions

1. Place in the bottom of the crockpot: olive oil, butter, garlic powder and parsley, onion powder, sriracha sauce chicken bouillon, and milk.
2. Pour in the macaroni and cheese and stir well.
3. Cook 1 ½ hours on low. Thirty minutes before it's done top with the bread crumbs.

Kale Pesto Risotto

Ingredients

- 2 tablespoons extra virgin olive oil
- 1 shallot, chopped
- 1 garlic clove, minced
- 4 kale leaves, chopped
- 1 cup wild rice
- 2 tablespoons pesto sauce
- ¼ cup dry white wine
- 2 cups chicken stock
- Salt and pepper to taste

Directions:

1. Heat the oil in a saucepan and stir in the shallot, garlic, and the kale. Cook for 2 minutes until softened.
2. Stir in the rice and cook for 2 additional minutes then add the pesto sauce, wine and stock, then season with salt and pepper.

3. Cook on low heat for 25-30 minutes until thickened and creamy.
4. Serve the risotto warm.

Chile

Ingredients:

- 2 medium unpeeled white or red potatoes (about 10 oz), cut into 1/2-inch cubes
- 1 medium onion, chopped (1/2 cup)
- 1 small bell pepper (any color), chopped (1/2 cup)
- 1 can (15 oz) chickpeas (garbanzo beans), drained, rinsed
- 1 can (15 oz) kidney beans, drained, rinsed
- 2 cans (14.5 oz each) organic diced tomatoes, undrained
- 1 can (8 oz) organic tomato sauce
- 1 tablespoon chili powder
- 1 teaspoon ground cumin
- 1 medium zucchini, cut into 1/2-inch slices

Directions:

1. In 4-quart Dutch oven, place all ingredients except zucchini; stir well. Heat to boiling over high heat, stirring occasionally; reduce heat. Cover; simmer 10 minutes.
2. Stir in zucchini. Cover; cook 5 to 7 minutes longer, stirring occasionally, until potatoes and zucchini are tender when pierced with fork.

Oven-Roasted Potatoes and Vegetables

Ingredients:

- 2 ½ cups refrigerated new potato wedges (from 1 lb 4-oz bag)
- 1 medium red bell pepper, cut into 1-inch pieces
- 1 small zucchini, cut into 1/2-inch pieces
- 4 oz fresh whole mushrooms, quartered (about 1 cup)
- 2 teaspoons olive oil
- ½ teaspoon dried Italian seasoning
- ¼ teaspoon garlic salt

Directions:

1. Heat oven to 450°F. Spray 15x10x1-inch pan with cooking spray. In large bowl, toss all ingredients to coat. Spread evenly in pan.
2. Bake 15 to 20 minutes, stirring once halfway through baking time, until vegetables are tender and lightly browned.

Roasted Rosemary-Onion Potatoes

Ingredients:

- 4 medium potatoes (1 1/3 pounds)
- 1 small onion, finely chopped (1/4 cup)
- 2 tablespoons olive or vegetable oil
- 2 tablespoons chopped fresh rosemary leaves or 2 teaspoons dried rosemary leaves
- 1 teaspoon chopped fresh thyme leaves or 1/4 teaspoon dried thyme leaves
- ¼ teaspoon salt
- 1/8 teaspoon pepper

Directions:

1. Heat oven to 450°F. Grease jelly roll pan, 15 1/2x10 1/2x1 inch. Cut potatoes into 1-inch chunks.
2. Mix remaining ingredients in large bowl. Add potatoes; toss to coat. Spread potatoes in single layer in pan.
3. Bake uncovered 20 to 25 minutes, turning occasionally, until potatoes are light brown and tender when pierced with fork.

Spiced Eggplant Stew

Ingredients

- 2 tablespoons extra virgin olive oil
- 2 shallots, chopped
- 4 garlic cloves, minced
- 1 carrot, diced 1 parsnip, diced
- 1 turnip, peeled and diced
- 2 large eggplants, cubed
- ½ teaspoon cumin powder
- ¼ teaspoon chili powder
- ¼ teaspoon coriander powder
- 2 cups diced tomatoes
- 1 bay leaf
- 1 cup vegetable stock
- Salt and pepper for taste

Directions

1. Heat the oil in a saucepan and stir in the shallots, garlic, carrot, parsnip and turnip.
2. Add the eggplants as well. Cook for 5 minutes then add the spices, tomatoes, bay leaf and stock, as well as salt and pepper.

3. Cook on low heat for 30 minutes.
4. Serve the stew warm and fresh.

Chapter 11: Desserts

Creamy Fruit Tarts

Ingredients:

- 1 cup Bisquick mix
- 2 tablespoons sugar
- 1 tablespoon butter or margarine, softened
- 2 packages (3 ounces each) cream cheese, softened
- ¼ cup sugar or 2 tablespoons of Splenda
- ¼ cup sour cream
- 1 ½ cups assorted sliced fresh fruit or berries
- 1/3 cup apple jelly, melted

Directions:

1. Heat oven to 375°F. Mix Bisquick, 2 tablespoons sugar, the butter and 1 package cream cheese in small bowl until dough forms a ball.
2. Divide dough into 6 parts. Press each part dough on bottom and 3/4 inch up side in each of 6 tart pans, 4 1/4 x 1 inch, or 10-ounce custard cups. Place on cookie sheet.
3. Bake 10 to 12 minutes or until light brown. Cool in pans on wire rack, about 30 minutes. Remove tart shells from pans.
4. Beat remaining package cream cheese, 1/4 cup sugar and the sour cream until smooth. Spoon into tart shells, spreading over bottoms. Top each with about 1/4 cup fruit. Brush with jelly.

Strawberry and Peach Cream Trifle

Ingredients

- 2 packages (4-serving size each) vanilla pudding and pie filling mix, (not instant)
- 3 cups milk
- 1 ½ quarts (6 cups) strawberries, sliced
- 1 large fresh peach, peeled and cubed
- ¼ cup sugar or 2 tablespoons of Splenda
- 1 package (16 ounces) frozen pound cake loaf
- ¼ cup peach or strawberry preserves
- ¼ cup amaretto or orange juice
- 1 cup whipping (heavy) cream
- ¼ cup slivered almonds, toasted
- 2 large fresh peaches, peeled and sliced

Directions

1. Make pudding mix as directed on package for pudding, using 3 cups milk. Place plastic wrap directly on top of pudding. Refrigerate at least 2 hours until chilled.
2. Mix strawberries, cubed peach and sugar. Let stand at room temperature 15 minutes.
3. Cut pound cake horizontally in half. Spread preserves over bottom half. Top with top half. Cut into 18 slices. Drizzle with amaretto. Place 9 slices in 3- to 4-quart straight-sided glass bowl. Spoon half of strawberry mixture over cake.
4. Beat whipping cream in chilled small bowl with electric mixer on high speed until stiff. Fold whipped cream into pudding. Spoon half of pudding mixture over strawberries. Repeat layers with remaining cake, strawberry mixture and pudding mixture. Refrigerate at least 2 hours.
5. Just before serving, sprinkle with almonds. Top with sliced peaches.

Vanilla Bean Pudding

Ingredients

- 2 ½ cups
- 2% reduced-fat milk
- 1 vanilla bean, split lengthwise
- ¾ cup sugar or 6 tablespoons Splenda
- 3 tablespoons cornstarch
- 1/8 teaspoon salt
- ¼ cup half-and-half
- 2 large egg yolks
- 4 teaspoons butter

Directions

1. Place milk in a medium, heavy saucepan. Scrape seeds from vanilla bean; add seeds and bean to milk. Bring to a boil.
2. Combine sugar, cornstarch, and salt in a large bowl, stirring well. Combine half-and-half and egg yolks, stirring well. Stir egg yolk mixture into sugar mixture. Gradually add half of hot milk to sugar mixture, stirring constantly with a whisk. Return hot milk mixture to pan; bring to a boil. Cook 1 minute, stirring constantly with a whisk. Remove from heat. Add butter, stirring until melted. Remove vanilla bean; discard.
3. Spoon pudding into a bowl. Place bowl in a large ice-filled bowl for 15 minutes or until pudding cools, stirring occasionally. Cover surface of pudding with plastic wrap; chill.

Baked Apples w/ Walnuts & Honey

Ingredients

- 4 medium sized apples
- 1 cup finely chopped walnuts
- 1 tablespoon honey
- 1 egg white
- 1 teaspoon vanilla extract
- zest of a half of lemon
- pinch of salt

Directions

1. Preheat the oven at 350 degrees.
2. Whip the egg white with the salt. the salt to stiff peaks, add the honey and beat until mixed. Fold in lemon zest, vanilla and walnuts.
3. Cut apples in pieces and core them. Lay the apples skin side down on a baking dish and fill the middle with the mixture. Bake for 40-45 minutes until apples are soft and filling crisps on top. Serve immediately.

Apricot Galette

Ingredients

- 1 ½ cups whole wheat flour
- 1 pinch salt
- ¼ teaspoon baking powder
- ½ cup coconut oil, melted
- 2 tablespoons cold water
- 1 ½ pounds apricots, halved
- 3 tablespoons raw honey
- ½ teaspoon cinnamon powder

Directions

1. Mix the flour, salt, baking powder, oil and cold water in a bowl and mix until a dough forms.
2. Transfer the dough on a floured working surface and knead it quickly to form it into a dough.
3. Roll the dough into a thin round sheet, giving it a round shape.
4. Place the apricots in the center of the dough and drizzle with honey.
5. Sprinkle with cinnamon then wrap the edges of the dough over the apricots, leaving the center exposed.
6. Bake in the preheated oven at 350F for 30 minutes.
7. Serve the galette chilled.

Carrot-Pineapple Muffins

Ingredients

- 2 cups almond flour
- 2 whisked eggs
- 1 tablespoon coconut flour
- ½ cup peeled grated carrots
- ¾ cup chopped fresh pineapple
- ¼ cup melted raw honey
- ¼ cup melted coconut oil
- 1 teaspoon cinnamon
- ½ teaspoon baking soda
- ½ teaspoon sea salt
- ¼ teaspoon allspice
- 1/8 teaspoon cloves

Directions

1. Preheat the oven at 350 degrees.

2. In a mixing bowl combine dry ingredients. In another mixing bowl combine wet ingredients. Add wet ingredients to dry And stir until combined.
3. Bake for 40-45 minutes until apples are soft and filling crisps on top. Serve immediately.

Banana Bread

Ingredients

- 2 cups almond flour
- 2 tablespoons coconut flour
- 2 whisked eggs (include yolk)
- 3 mashed ripe bananas
- ¼ cup melted raw honey
- ¼ cup melted coconut oil
- 1 teaspoon vanilla extract
- 1 teaspoon cinnamon
- ¾ teaspoon baking soda
- ½ teaspoon sea salt

Directions

1. Preheat the oven at 350 degrees.
2. In mixing bowl combine dry ingredients (Almond flour, coconut flour, spices, baking soda and sea salt). In another bowl combine wet ingredients (eggs, honey, coconut oil, vanilla extract). Add wet ingredients to dry ingredients and stir until combined. Add mashed bananas and mix together.
3. Place in a greased (non-stick cooking spray 9x5 loaf pan) and bake 40- 45 min depending on oven.

Moroccan Spiced Orange Salad

Ingredients

- 6 oranges, cut into segments
- 1 teaspoon lemon juice
- ¼ teaspoon cinnamon powder
- ¼ teaspoon ground ginger
- 1 teaspoon orange zest
- 2 tablespoons sliced almonds

Directions

1. Combine the orange segments, lemon juice, cinnamon, ginger, orange zest and almonds in a bowl.
2. Serve immediately.

Blackberry Cobbler

Ingredients

- 1 ½ pounds fresh blackberries
- 1 tablespoon lemon juice
- ¼ cup maple syrup
- 1 tablespoon cornstarch
- ¼ teaspoon ground ginger
- 1 cup whole wheat flour
- 1 cup rolled oats
- 2 tablespoons raw honey
- ¼ cup coconut oil, melted

Directions

1. Combine the blackberries, lemon juice, maple syrup, cornstarch and ginger in a deep dish baking pan.
2. For the topping, combine the wheat flour, oats, honey and coconut oil in a bowl and mix well.
3. Spread this mixture over the blackberries and bake in the preheated oven at 350F for 35-40 minutes until the topping is golden brown and crisp.
4. Serve chilled.

Raspberry Tarts

Ingredients

- 1 cup/ 250 ml milk
- ½ vanilla bean, halved lengthwise and seeds scraped
- 3 egg yolks
- ¼ cup/ 55 g sugar
- 2 tablespoons flour
- 1 tablespoon framboise (raspberry liqueur)
- ¼ cup heavy cream
- 1 pound/ 450 g fresh raspberries
- 1 (9-inch/ 23 cm) prepared baked cookie crust

Directions

1. Put the milk in a saucepan. Split the vanilla bean, scraping the seeds into the milk, then drop in the pot. Heat to a simmer, remove from heat, cover, and set to infuse 10 minutes.
2. In bowl using an electric mixer, beat the yolks with the sugar until pale. Beat in the flour. Pull the vanilla bean from the milk and whisk the milk gradually into the egg mixture. Pour back into the saucepan, bring to a boil, and cook 1 minute. Remove from the heat and stir in the framboise. Strain into a bowl, cover with plastic wrap,

and set aside to cool. When chilled, whip the cream and gently fold it in.
3. Spread the pastry cream evenly in the base of the prepared cookie crust. Arrange the berries neatly over top.

Grilled Peaches with Yogurt

Ingredients

- 2 large peaches, halved and pitted
- 2 tablespoons raw honey
- ½ teaspoon cinnamon powder
- 1 cup low fat plain yogurt
- ¼ cup sliced almonds

Directions

1. Drizzle the peach halves with honey and sprinkle with cinnamon powder.
2. Heat a grill pan over medium flame and place the peaches on the grill.
3. Cook until browned then place on serving plates.
4. Top with yogurt and almond slices and serve right away.

Conclusion

I had a lot of goals when I set out to write this book, but the most important of these was to shed light on the Gout and its management through an effective clean eating diet.

You have one life to live. If you have Gout, it is not a death sentence, but rather, a wake-up call for you to take better care of yourself. Think of it as a blessing in disguise. You are going to have to make some changes. That's it. Diet is one of those things that is under our control.

Whether you need to take medicine for gout or not you should ensure that you follow these simple rules of thumb:

- Limit alcoholic beverages and drinks sweetened with fruit sugar (fructose).
- Drink plenty of nonalcoholic beverages, especially water.
- Limit intake of foods high in purines, such as red meat, organ meats and seafood.
- Exercise regularly and lose weight. Keeping your body at a healthy weight reduces your risk of gout.

I hope you enjoyed this book and found it useful. Now that you have a basic understanding of gout and some its causes and remedies coupled with 'clean' gout friendly fair, I want you to act on what you have learned and BEAT gout into your past, where it belongs.

You are what you eat!

www.ingramcontent.com/pod-product-compliance
Lightning Source LLC
Chambersburg PA
CBHW061158180526
45170CB00002B/856